A Caregiver's
Journey

A Caregiver's Journey

Finding Your Way

Karen L. Twichell

Writers Club Press

San Jose New York Lincoln Shanghai

A Caregiver's Journey
Finding Your Way

Writers Club Press
an imprint of iUniverse.com, Inc.

For information address:
iUniverse.com, Inc.
5220 S 16th, Ste. 200
Lincoln, NE 68512
www.iuniverse.com

ISBN: 0-595-16835-3

Printed in the United States of America

With love to Linda Thiel for her quiet courage, and JoAnne George for her graceful strength, and Bruce Twichell, who was willing to share me during the most difficult of times. And in memory of Michael Koepke, Marian Koepke and Edwin Koepke.

With the utmost respect to the millions of caregivers worldwide who give of themselves to make the lives of their loved ones somehow better.

"Man is not born to solve the problems of the universe, but to find out what he has to do…within the limits of his comprehension."

Johann von Goethe

Contents

Personal Stories

Foreword

A Caregiver's Journey is powerful, truthful and most of all, helpful. Karen Twichell knows that nothing measures the depth of our humanity more than our ability to give love and care to those around us. Few experiences are more meaningful or more demanding. Take some time to read this book and you'll be better prepared when life gives you the ultimate responsibility. Beautifully written and carefully observed, *A Caregiver's Journey* should become an indispensable part of every adult's library.

T. Jefferson Parker, former caregiver and author of *Red Light*

Acknowledgements

Thank you to Linda, JoAnne and Bruce for letting me share their lives and their very personal stories.

Thank you to the many caregivers who have opened their hearts to me and allowed me to join them for a little while on their respective journeys.

Thank you to Laura Elek, valued friend and author who tirelessly listened and read my manuscript over and over.

Thank you to Ann Brandt and Dessa Reed, authors/friends, who never let me give up.

Thank you to Shannon and John Tullius for making the Maui Writers Conference available to those of us who have a dream and need to share it with others. You made the difference.

Thank you to the many family members and friends who supported this project from the beginning and gave me a reason to see it through.

And thank you to the professionals who gave me their knowledge and their time to ensure accuracy in my work.

WHAT OTHERS ARE SAYING ABOUT THIS BOOK

"I strongly recommend this book to all friends and family members whose lives have been touched by serious illness. The advice and comfort offered by Ms. Twichell is invaluable because she's been there and grown through the personal challenges and tragedies." Linda Bosserman, M.D., Medical Oncology and Hematology.

"A Caregiver's Journey is indispensable for the people often forgotten when illness strikes." Kathy Pearson, RN, CNS, AOCN, Oncology Clinical Nurse Specialist

"A Caregiver's Journey touches the heart, presenting both common sense and empathy through personal stories never before offered on the subject of serious illness." Reverend James Covey, Executive Director, Inland Hospice Association

Chapter 1

When You Hurt, I Hurt

*The entire sum of existence is the magic
of being needed by just one person.*

Vi Putnam

This year well over one million Americans will be diagnosed with cancer. For each new patient there will be someone introduced to the world of caregiving. Add to this number thousands of AIDS, stroke, heart disease and Alzheimer's cases and you discover that there is an entire community of caregivers who have many of the same fears and concerns as the patients they care about.

Caregiving is a responsibility no one wants. It creates a horrible, helpless feeling. It tests your strength, your courage and your faith. It makes you feel like a failure because you can't cure the disease or ease the pain. It makes you hate God and the medical profession because they won't make your patient well. It makes you angry and sad and so afraid of what will happen next. It makes you want to do everything today because you are afraid tomorrow will not come.

Patients receive the initial diagnosis and immediately become the focus of attention by their medical team and by their families. They are bombarded with information about their disease, about treatment and about support groups. They are offered books and pamphlets and videos and group sessions. But who is there to help the caregiver? Families dealing with life-threatening illnesses often feel isolated from the rest of the world. There is little information available about families coping with illness on a day-to-day basis. It is not my intent to diminish in any way the horror faced by the patient, but to address the specific concerns of the caregiver. The spirits of the most loving and courageous people can be broken by the anguish of a serious illness.

A Caregiver's Journey is a book for and about caregivers. The text offers some practical guidance to individuals who suddenly find themselves in the role of caregiver, as well as true stories that serve to share experiences that will help the readers understand that they are not alone. Caregivers often feel they must be strong at all times, never show fear, always smile. The emotions that consume a caregiver are every bit as real as those that grip the patient. Caregivers will take comfort in knowing the fears and frustrations they feel are shared by millions of others. The following chapters will address such issues as the initial diagnosis, communication, physical, emotional and spiritual concerns, getting help, hostile patients and caregivers, and taking care of yourself.

This book is dedicated to those who have held the hand of a dying loved one or cried at the bedside of a sister whose body has been ravaged by chemotherapy or radiation. It is dedicated to those who have waited by the phone for the results of yet another procedure, or simply listened with their hearts to someone going through similar experiences.

At some point in our lives, most of us become caregivers in one way or another. It may be for a brief time following an accident or surgery until a patient is well. It may be for months or years resulting in the death of the patient. It is a world full of sadness and fear. It is heart wrenching. It is also necessary and rewarding. This book is dedicated to you.

Chapter 2

Hearing the News

*Everyday...life confronts us with new problems to be
solved which force us to adjust our old programs accordingly.*

Dr. Ann Faraday

The diagnosis of a life-threatening disease brings feelings of shock, fear and often denial. Each patient is different and will express his or her feelings differently. Loved ones hearing about this diagnosis will experience many of the same emotions. The patient most often hears the news from the attending physician. The loved one, who will soon become a caregiver, hears it from the patient, who may or may not have had time to really absorb the information. Hearing the initial diagnosis can be devastating. For the caregiver, as for the patient, this event marks the beginning of a journey that neither wants to take.

By listening carefully to what the patient is saying, a caregiver can begin to determine what makes the patient most able to deal with the diagnosis. Some patients want to read everything available about their disease and treatment options as fast as they can. Some just want to be told where to be and when for treatments. Still others want to discuss their illnesses, others don't. It is important for the caregiver to be sensitive to the feelings of the patient. It is also important, however, to remember that caregivers, like patients, deal differently with each situation. For some it is important to "do something" right away. It may be searching the Internet for information, or going to the library for books about a specific disease. Others may want to comfort the patient, yet don't always know how to go about it. Then there are those who won't be able to deal with the situation at all and will withdraw completely. Often what is most needed is someone who will simply listen while feelings are expressed. Deciding how to tell a loved one about the diagnosis is likely the first of many difficult decisions a patient will have to make. It means that a loved one has to say out loud, for perhaps the first time, that his or her life is being threatened by disease.

The primary caregiver, after hearing the news, might be able to assist the patient with the task of informing other family members and friends. The caregiver might arrange an informal meeting for special individuals where information about the diagnosis and what type of treatment is being planned can be presented. This is a good time to let others know ways in which they may be helpful in the weeks and months ahead. Give them a chance to express their feelings and ask questions. This is also an opportune time to set up an information system that removes the burden from the patient and the primary caregiver of having to repeat information in response to inquiries from caring individuals. Keeping this communication system intact throughout the treatment will ensure that, as needs change or additional assistance is required, it's not necessary to start over. This core group is also the group that will be there for celebrations throughout the various stages of treatment.

"Fix yourself a stiff drink…"

When my brother was ill and suspected something serious might be wrong, he entrusted his secret to me. This was a heavy burden that eventually came to light when he was hospitalized. After he died, my sisters and I promised we would never keep health secrets from one another.

In July 1995, my younger sister, 48, and I received a letter on the same day from our older sister, 55. "I was going to call you both," the letter began, "but I decided to take the coward's way out and do it by mail." I remember sitting down to read the letter. I've never thought of JoAnne as being cowardly about anything and I believe she chose to tell us about her breast cancer diagnosis this way to give us time to absorb what she was saying. She is a very methodical person who would want to have as much information as she could before she wrote to us and so the letter contained all the details about the surgery schedule, who the doctors were and what to expect after the surgery. Long before she gets emotional, she gets organized and that is her way of dealing with a crisis. I am very much like her in this respect. I read the letter several times, absorbing each detail, trying to deny the message. But the message was clear and the first of many tears began to flow. The three of us talked on the phone that night and continued to talk openly throughout her treatment.

The following February, I came home from work to a message on my answering machine from my younger sister, Linda. "Fix yourself a stiff drink and call me," she said. The week before she had minor surgery for a small growth in her colon thought to be benign. The initial diagnosis was wrong. She had colon cancer. JoAnne was completing her chemotherapy and radiation treatments. Just four months earlier my mother died within weeks of her diagnosis of pancreatic cancer. Now, in the same week my husband was diagnosed with prostate cancer, my little sister was also stricken. I did fix that stiff drink and listened while she read the lab report to me. She was alone and I wanted to go to her and hold her. She said she was okay and needed some time. When I got off the phone, I cried my heart out while my husband held me and cried too. Then I took a deep breath and called my other sister and we cried again.

Was it any easier to hear the news by phone or by letter? This kind of news is never easy to hear. Let the patient decide how to share the diagnosis and then support the patient in that choice as you begin to support him or her in dealing with the reality of the prognosis.

NOTES:
Things I can do right away:

_____
_____
_____
_____
_____
_____
_____

My Core Support Group:

_____
_____
_____
_____
_____
_____
_____
_____
_____
_____
_____
_____
_____

Chapter 3

Listening, Talking

*Just be what you are and speak from your guts
and heart-it's all a man has.*

Hubert H. Humphrey

Candor and openness between patient and caregiver can keep imagin-
ings from growing into deep fears. Mutual confrontation of these fears
helps to keep them under control. When serious illness strikes, the
entire family is impacted. One of the greatest gifts you can offer is to be
a good listener. Listen to what is said and how it is said; learn to read
between the lines. Learn to feel comfortable when there is a lull in the
conversation. Silences help us focus our thoughts. Don't feel you have to
say something. Also remember that patients do not always want to
think or talk about their illnesses. Let them take the lead. Being there for
them and simply being you is often just what they need. At the same
time, it is important that you, as the caregiver, share your feelings, concerns and fears with the patient. Be careful not to use trite expressions
("…everything will be fine"). The message you convey is "don't tell me
you don't feel good". It's much better to say, "I'm sorry you don't feel
well. I'm glad to be here for you". This can open an entirely new kind of
dialog that will ultimately make both of you more comfortable having
these discussions. To open a conversation about serious illness, select a
time and place conducive to such a discussion. Make sure there is suffi-
cient time to have this conversation without interruption. A private area
in the comfort of one's own home can put both you and the patient at

ease. Make sure the patient knows you are available to discuss this uncomfortable topic at any time and let him decide when he wants to talk. At a time when so many decisions are no longer within the patient's control, he will appreciate retaining control over this issue. Be realistic about your expectations during these discussions. People communicate in different ways. Some are more open than others. Some people have never talked about their feelings. This pattern is not likely to change just because they are ill. It is especially important to realize the patient is not necessarily looking for advice, but simply wants support and understanding.

For both the caregiver and the patient, writing about feelings, rather than talking about them, may be more comfortable. Accept that either is fine and be available to read as well as talk if invited. Sharing your own writings with other caregivers can also be very therapeutic.

Caregivers need to understand that patients aren't always right and shouldn't necessarily get their way. We tend to feel guilty that they are the sick ones and we aren't, so we often do more than is really good for the patient. Continue to keep the lines of communication open. It is all right to ask a patient to do things that will make your caregiving responsibilities more manageable. You might suggest purchasing a new bed that would allow you to assist the patient more easily, or ask to be given a little more notice when the pain begins. Little things like these will ultimately make life easier for both the patient and the caregiver. It is extremely important for the patient to continue to make as many of his own decisions as possible. Taking away that privilege undermines the patient's feelings of self control. It is the patient's body, in most cases, that is ill, not his brain. Don't treat your patient as though he can no longer think.

Sometimes a Stranger

Darlene had come to the cancer resource library to obtain some information on ovarian cancer for a friend who had just had surgery, she said. But I think Darlene just wanted to talk to someone. Her young husband was fighting melanoma, a serious form of skin cancer. It had spread to his lymph nodes. She didn't want to talk to a friend, family or doctor. She simply needed to talk to someone who wasn't tired of hearing about it. She told me she had two small children. She is terrified of what might happen to her husband and then to the family. Darlene believes she is a rotten mom because she doesn't have time to go to every soccer game or read a story every night. She feels she isn't being strong if she cries or gets tired. In fact, Darlene is a very strong young woman and needed a stranger to tell her so. I did.

An Apple Pie

When Betty came in for her shift in the library, I was getting ready to leave. She told me her son, 43 years old, had been diagnosed with a malignant brain tumor six weeks before and she wasn't sure she could continue her volunteer work. I had never met this woman before. She told me her son was about to begin an experimental treatment program. She was praying it would save his life. She had baked him an apple pie that morning because she just didn't know what else to do. My own brother died at the age of 45 of a brain tumor. I listened, tried to be encouraging, left my shift and cried again for my brother who had died ten years before and for her son who I didn't even know.

Games–Anytime!

Todd tells the story of his wife, Erin who was dying of breast cancer. They knew her life was being measured in days and weeks, perhaps months at this time. There were good days and bad days, good nights and bad nights. They made an agreement not to waste any of the good days or nights. Erin was an avid Scrabble player and would frequently wake Todd at 2 or 3 a.m. and ask him to set up the board and they would play for hours. These are some of Todd's fondest memories. They would play and they would talk. While they played, they would talk about good things, not about the disease or death. Todd says he never could beat Erin at Scrabble, even when she was near the end and taking stronger medications! He now plays Scrabble with his two young children and they talk about the good times with their mommy.

More than Coincidence

JoAnne and I arrived early at the Race for the Cure in Newport Beach, California. We had just visited the survivor booth where JoAnne picked up her traditional pink survivor visor. As we walked away, a young woman approached us and asked JoAnne if she could ask her some questions. I continued to visit the booths while they talked. Tammy had been diagnosed with breast cancer only that week. Her mother had died from the same disease only two years before. It amazed me then, and it amazes me now that out of some 14,000 participants on that day, Tammy chose to talk to my sister. What is so amazing is that, as it turned out, Tammy was being treated at the same hospital and had the same oncologist as JoAnne. This race took place 50 miles from where that hospital is located!

During the brief time Tammy and JoAnne spent together, JoAnne was able to assure Tammy that she was being treated at a first class cancer care center by an exceptional medical team. They bonded instantly. JoAnne followed her progress from her first treatment to her last and they became friends. I do not know how much of a family support system Tammy had, but I know from watching the survivors in action, that a fellow survivor is a critical part of the caregiving team. I was proud to watch my sister in action, as I have many times since that day when some mysterious coincidence brought JoAnne and Tammy together in a crowd of thousands.

A Little Sensitivity, Please

Wouldn't you think everyone from the receptionist to the oncologist dealing with cancer patients would be particularly caring and sensitive? By the very nature of their chosen professions, these are the people we think we can count on to say the right thing at the right time when we lay people are often struggling to come up with the right response.

I recently witnessed an incident in an oncologist's office which made me realize this is not a fair assumption. A gentleman came out of the inner office having just completed his chemotherapy treatment. His skin was pale and he appeared fatigued. He told the receptionist he would see her next week, as he had every Friday for the past seven months. He said he felt as though he lived in that office. I was sure that her response would be something encouraging such as, "You'll soon be through your treatments and we'll miss seeing you." Instead, she didn't even look up from what she was doing and in a dull tone of voice replied, "Me too, I know just how you feel. Sometimes I feel like I'm just a part of the furniture in here." Unless she had been going through the treatment he was enduring, she couldn't possibly have known how he felt. Her incredibly insensitive comment reminded me, as a caregiver, to choose my words with caution so I never appear so insensitive to those I love.

NOTES
Things I want to talk about when the time is right:

_____

_____

_____

_____

_____

_____

_____

_____

_____

_____

I'm more comfortable expressing my feelings in writing:

_____

_____

_____

_____

_____

_____

_____

_____

_____

_____

_____

Chapter 4

Dealing with Doctors

A problem adequately stated is a problem well on its way to being solved.

R. Buckminster Fuller

Open communication between patient, caregiver and the medical team is critical to the health and recovery of the patient and to the mental well being of both the patient and the caregiver. Much frustration exists because caregivers often do not know how to ask questions in a way that will result in satisfactory answers.

We all want to be viewed as ideal patients and often have a reluctance to "bother the doctor" or "take too much of the doctor's time." We have experienced today's average doctor's appointment at seven minutes, as compared to 20 minutes only ten years ago.

In most cases, there is more than one doctor involved with a serious illness or injury. Often, there is also a team of nurses, social workers, or hospice personnel.

Begin by choosing doctors who make you and your patient comfortable. Many of us feel that we are "assigned" a doctor and have no options. This is usually not the case. If you find you have different attitudes toward treatment or how decisions are made, perhaps you are not compatible and you should request another physician. You will be spending a lot of time with this medical team and need to be able to focus on medical care, not personality conflicts.

Some general guidelines for clear communication with your medical team are:

- Write down your questions as you think of them between visits. Write them clearly or type them in large print. Just before the visit, arrange them in order of importance.

- When the doctor greets you with "how are you today?" hopefully your patient won't reply, "just fine", if you are preparing to ask questions about severe diarrhea. Instead, encourage your patient to say, "I'm generally feeling much better, but have had severe diarrhea for five days. I've tried this and that, and so far nothing helps."

- Begin asking questions at the start of the visit so the doctor is aware of what's going on right away and will be more patient than if you wait until the end of the session.

- After you ask your questions, be sure you are listening to the answers. Write the answers down if you don't think you will remember them.

- If you have articles from the Internet or magazines which you want to discuss, don't walk into the doctor's office with 20 pages and expect him to read and/or comment on them. Summarize by saying, "I read about a trial program on the Internet for the treatment of lymphoma (for instance). Is this something we could consider?" If the doctor asks you to leave the information, that's fine, but don't push it on him.

- It's a good thing to read and do research on your own, but caution must be exercised with the abundance of available information; it may not all be trustworthy.

- You may not always know exactly what to ask. Don't be too timid to ask the doctor if there's anything else you should be asking.

- Doctors are often reluctant to give a prognosis on life expectancy, particularly to the caregiver. You might approach the question by mentioning statistics you have read and ask the doctor if he agrees that they are credible. Remember, though, that they are only statistics and every day we meet people who have belied the statistics of their particular disease.

NOTES

Questions I want to ask the doctor or nurse

_____

_____

_____

_____

_____

_____

_____

_____

_____

_____

_____

Articles from the newspaper, magazines or Internet I want to take to the doctor:

_____

_____

_____

_____

_____

_____

_____

_____

_____

_____

_____

Chapter 5

Treatment Journal

What the world really needs is more love and less paperwork.

Pearl Bailey

One of the most valuable tools a caregiver can use is a treatment journal. This is the journal the patient would keep if not so exhausted by the entire experience of the illness. Keeping meticulous records from the very beginning of the treatment can make the months ahead much easier on the patient and on you, the caregiver. Your journal can be a favorite notebook or a calendar with lots of room to write. Make sure you have lots of space for entries, as this journal will grow more rapidly than you can imagine. You will need lots of sections you can easily identify to get you to the correct information quickly when you need it. The first thing you need to enter into your notebook is your name, address and phone number with a notation that this is a very valuable notebook and if found, please return.

Begin by creating a section of detailed information about each of the patient's doctors. Make it clear if the doctor is the oncologist or the urologist or cardiologist. There will be many doctors working together when a patient is seriously ill. You may chose to switch doctors from time to time, and a notation should be made when that occurs. Include names, addresses and phone numbers for each doctor as well as identification numbers, if needed for insurance purposes. It can also be helpful to jot down names of nurses and front office personnel for future use when making appointments.

Although you already have a personal telephone directory, add a section to your journal that includes the phone numbers of all of the people you might want to call from a doctor's office or the hospital. This would include family members, friends, support organizations and pharmacies. Make a special notation of who should be called in case of an emergency.

Time and time again you will be asked to fill out forms regarding the medical history of the patient. The first time you do this, ask for a copy of it and put it in your journal. Then, each time you are asked again, you simply have to copy the information without looking up insurance numbers, birth dates, test date information and so on. Use caution here, however, checking periodically to make certain your information is accurate. Update the information by making changes in red ink. Taking the time to do a thorough medical history on your patient at the beginning will make repeat requests less bothersome and be useful many times. It is essential you have details at your fingertips about every aspect of the disease and the treatment. Each new doctor you see will want exact dates of such things as heart attacks, biopsies, blood work, CAT scans, and every other aspect of your treatment. If you have it all written in your journal, you won't have to guess. You will also be assisting the doctor in providing better care.

Oftentimes your patient will begin a particular type of treatment; then it will be decided that something else is preferable. Knowing what treatment was started and on what date it was stopped is extremely valuable information.

While it may seem like a formidable task, making notations about each and every medication prescribed is essential. Make columns to record who prescribed the medication, when the patient started to take it, how well it was tolerated, if it was successful and when it was stopped. Note any allergic reactions. In the course of treatment, many doctors will come and go and may prescribe something your patient has already taken. You can save time, money and aggravation by having medication information readily available whenever you are in a doctor's office or the hospital. Using the same pharmacy for all prescriptions can be beneficial as well, as the pharmacy will have all your patient's records in one place. Also, the pharmacist is more likely to notice a conflict in medications. Note any over-the-counter medications your patient is taking, such as vitamins and antacids as there may be a conflict with prescribed medications.

Allocate a section of your journal for questions you would like to ask the doctors during your next visit. None of us can remember on demand what it was we meant to ask, so write it down and then you can forget about it until you are in the doctor's office for the next visit. Don't cross a question off your list until you are completely satisfied with the answer. Most doctors appreciate your interest and are happy to answer questions or, refer you to someone else.

The final section of your journal should include blank pages which can be used to write down personal thoughts. This can be a very therapeutic exercise. There are many times when you will be sitting in the waiting room over the next few months while your patient is receiving care. Sometimes it helps to talk to others; sometimes it helps to write down how YOU are feeling.

NOTES

I'll set up my treatment journal this week. To do this I need the following items:

_____

_____

_____

_____

_____

_____

_____

_____

_____

_____

_____

_____

_____

_____

Chapter 6

Physical Issues

*She didn't talk to me or try to tell me everything was
all right because she knew it wasn't. She stayed with me and
relief came, not because of what she did but because she was there.*

Scott Burton,
Cancer Survivor and
Author

A Life in the
Balance

Providing effective physical care in the most comfortable way possible begins with learning about the specific challenges that your patient faces with his particular illness. Medical care is the most tangible part of your patient's recovery and the best way to get started is to learn everything you can about the disease and the treatment plan. Learn what the options are and their possible side effects. Discuss these options with the patient if he is willing and support his decision, even if it's not the one you would have chosen. Determine how to make your patient as comfortable as possible during his treatment. You must also recognize that regardless of how good you are as a caregiver, the treatment may fail.

While some general guidelines for caring for the ill apply in all cases, some are unique to the particular disease. A patient with breast cancer, for example, may have a mastectomy and will require several weeks of recuperation. There will be drainage tubes and the incision will need special care. She will need assistance with physical therapy and, in many cases, will require radiation and chemotherapy. Whether or not to have breast reconstruction is a very personal decision. Be sure that your patient knows what her options are and support her in her decision. Self-esteem can be an issue for breast cancer survivors. Remind her often of her wit, her personal accomplishments and how much she means to you.

Side effects vary widely depending on the illness. Remembering that most side effects are temporary can be very helpful to both the patient and the caregiver. Knowing that the diarrhea will stop one day and there will be a full head of hair again can be very encouraging. Knowing about the side effects and how to treat them is a major part of the caregiver's job. Some of the most common side effects that your patient might face as a result of chemotherapy, radiation, the nature of his particular illness or simply the anxiety of being ill could include the following:

- Diarrhea: Diarrhea is a condition of more frequent and more fluid bowel movements than usual. The bowel movements may be accompanied by cramps. Diarrhea can be caused by chemotherapy or radiation therapy, bacterial and viral infections, medications, surgery, anxiety and the growth of tumors. When diarrhea strikes your patient, try to encourage him to drink 8 to 12 glasses of clear liquid a day. Drinking more fluids will not worsen the diarrhea and will help prevent dehydration. Clear liquids eliminate overwork by the bowels and guard against irritation. Apple juice, peach or apricot nectar, tea or broth is recommended. Liquids should be served at room temperature to prevent muscle contractions caused by hot or cold liquids. When the patient is feeling better, foods low in roughage but high in protein, calories and potassium can gradually be added to his diet. Such foods include cottage cheese, eggs, baked or mashed potatoes, boiled white rice, bananas, macaroni, toast and peanut butter are some recommended foods. Small frequent meals are suggested rather than three large meals. Foods that should be avoided while the patient is dealing with diarrhea include fried or greasy foods, nuts, raw fruits and vegetables, spicy foods and alcohol. Milk and milk products should not be consumed during this time. If the diarrhea continues for more than a few days with more than six bowel movements per day, or there is blood in the stool, call the doctor. Also let the doctor know if your patient loses five or more pounds after the diarrhea starts. There are many diarrhea medications on the market from over-the-counter products to prescription drugs. The doctor will prescribe what is best for your patient depending on the symptoms exhibited.

- Fatigue: The fatigue often experienced by people with serious illnesses is described as an excessive whole-body tiredness that is not resolved by rest or sleep. Fatigue can have a profound negative impact on the quality of life and often interferes with the type of activities that make life enjoyable. As fatigue begins to interfere with what your patient can do for himself, you will begin to assume many of the tasks previously performed by the patient. These increased demands can lead to fatigue for you as a caregiver as well, and caution must be exercised to protect both of you from further fatigue. When fatigue sets in, it can be very helpful to keep a journal for the patient to identify the time of day when fatigue is greatest. This will help identify the contributing factors. Be alert for the signs of fatigue, such as tired eyes, stiff shoulders, decreased energy, inability to concentrate, decreased attention to personal appearance, impatience or sleepiness. When these signs appear, encourage the patient to rest to prevent an increase in fatigue. Help your patient learn to pace himself and to understand that this is just a temporary condition. While combating illness, the body requires more rest and more sleep. Plan ahead for naps and schedule activities to allow for rest periods. Encourage the patient to select the activities that are most important and let the others go or ask someone else to attend to them. Reassure your patient that this restructuring of his life is just for a short time and he will slowly get back to normal. As a caregiver, you can help by offering a well-balanced diet, providing eight glasses of liquid a day to prevent dehydration and supporting the idea of moderate exercise. Perhaps taking a walk together each morning would get the patient moving and would be good for you as well! You can protect the patient from fatigue by setting limits on visitors and phone calls, which can be exhausting. Don't force your patient to do more than he can comfortably manage. Let others help with meals, housework and errands. Promote frequent naps as long as they don't interfere with normal sleep patterns. Establish bedtime rituals to help both you and the patient fall asleep and enjoy a good night's rest.

- Hair Loss (also known as alopecia): This is the most visible side effect of cancer treatment and is often the most upsetting. As a caregiver, you can be very helpful in assisting your patient plan for the effects of chemotherapy as the drugs circulate throughout the body, destroying rapidly growing cells such as hair and the cells that line the mouth and gastrointestinal tract. Not all drugs cause hair loss. If hair loss does occur, it usually begins within two weeks of the start of treatment and gradually worsens over the next couple of months. Hair can begin to grow again even before therapy is complete. You can help ease the trauma of this side effect by encouraging your patient to purchase a wig or toupee in advance of his treatment. This early purchase of a wig provides a better texture and hair color match. Insurance companies will often cover the cost of a wig as part of the treatment plan. A little research in advance by the caregiver can alleviate questions about the financial impact to the patient. If the patient has long hair, a visit to a beauty salon for a short haircut in advance will make the hair loss less noticeable to both the patient and others. Prior to loss of the hair, encourage the use of gentle shampoos and soft brushes. Avoid hair coloring and permanents. Discourage the use of electric rollers, hair dryers and curling irons. Go shopping with the patient to purchase a few hats or scarves so that there are options each day. Most importantly, remind your patient that the hair almost always comes back. It may take 3 to 6 months, or it might come back while the patient is still in treatment. When it does come back, it might have a slightly different texture or color, or curl. Looking at a calendar and planning for the day when the wig or hairpiece will no longer be needed is a good reminder that this is a temporary condition. Patients often like their after-treatment hair better than they did their previous hair. There have been cases of caregivers shaving their heads in support of their patients. While you may not want to go that far, it would be a good idea not to complain about a bad-hair day during this time!

- Loss of Appetite: One of the most common side effects of chemotherapy, but it can also result from radiation therapy, stress and anxiety, depression and the illness itself. Unfortunately, appetite is lost just when your patient needs proper nourishment the most. Studies have shown that patients fighting life-threatening diseases need hundreds more calories and at least twice the amount of protein as healthy people do. Your patient must get enough nourishment to provide him with the strength and ability he needs to fight his disease. As a result of chemotherapy, your patient may lose all desire to eat as foods and liquids now have different tastes. Sweet foods sometimes lose their sweetness and proteins begin to taste bitter. Whatever the cause, loss of appetite is usually temporary and can be relieved within a few weeks. Caregivers can be of particular value during this time because the patient may be able to tolerate food more readily if prepared by others. If odors are too offensive when prepared in the home, arrangements might be made with a neighbor to do the preparation in their home for a brief period of time. Serving the meal cold or at room temperature to decrease its smell and taste might also help. By making the meal time a pleasant experience, the caregiver can encourage better eating by the patient. Prepare high calorie foods that are easily digested and try marinating meats in fruit juices or soy sauce to help improve the taste. Create a relaxed atmosphere and serve the meal in the most attractive way possible. This can become a discouraging process if the patient refuses to eat. Remember, however, that as a caregiver, you need and deserve a nicely prepared meal too. Asking in advance what the patient might like makes him a part of the meal planning process. If the patient can tolerate it and would enjoy a small glass of wine before meals, it may help to relax him and stimulate his taste buds. A 5 to 10-minute walk about half an hour before meals will also help to stimulate the appetite. Above all, encourage your patient to eat as much as he can manage, but do not force the issue. This pressure only creates anxiety, making it even more difficult to eat. Loss of appetite need not become the focus of the relationship between you and your partner.

- Nausea and Vomiting: Nausea is a feeling of stomach distress accompanied by an urge to throw up. Vomiting is throwing up. Nausea and vomiting can be temporary side effects of chemotherapy and radiation therapy. They can also be the result of an obstruction in the intestine, irritation of the gastrointestinal tract or brain tumors. Frequent vomiting can be dangerous because it can lead to dehydration or to inhaling foods or liquids. Every effort should be made to assist the patient in controlling nausea before vomiting starts. Vast improvements have been made in controlling nausea during chemotherapy treatments. Doctors and nurses are prepared to handle these side effects through the use of new and effective medications that can be given along with chemotherapy treatments. Before the first treatment is given, be optimistic and encourage your patient regarding the success of new anti-nausea drugs. Many patients experience nausea before they even begin their treatments because of the fear that has been planted in them and this is known as anticipatory nausea and vomiting. Some things that might help reduce the chance of suffering from nausea and vomiting before a scheduled treatment might include:

- maintaining a clear liquid diet one to 12 hours before treatment
- practicing behavioral techniques such as hypnosis, relaxation therapy, imagery or listening to your favorite music to help you relax.

During and after treatment, try:

- eating bland foods, such as crackers
- eating small amounts of food more frequently
- eating meals at room temperature or cooler
- keeping the house free of offensive odors
- seeking a relaxing atmosphere, reading a book or watching television.

As caregivers we, of course, want to please and want to help, but a word of caution here. We might be tempted to offer the patient's favorite foods to encourage him to eat. Yet, it is recommended that patients actually avoid their favorite foods when they are being treated with chemotherapy as they will often develop an aversion to that particular food and never really enjoy it again.

- Lymphedema: a medical term used to describe swelling caused by the buildup of fluid in soft tissues. This swelling develops because of a blockage of the lymphatic system. Lymphedema can result from radical surgical procedures with lymph node dissection or after an acute inflammation such as an infection in the limb. It usually involves the areas near the largest collection of lymph nodes such as the armpit, pelvic or groin areas. When the lymphatics are obstructed, a swelling in the arms or legs can result. Lymphedema can be acute or chronic. Acute lymphedema is a temporary condition that can happen after a surgical procedure or after an acute inflammation such as an infection to a limb. Cancer patients more often suffer chronic lymphedema. It can range from minor swelling and discomfort to grave disability and disfigurement. Chronic lymphedema is much more difficult to reverse than the acute variety because the more the limb swells the harder it is to drain the fluid adequately. People with chronic lymphedema are also more susceptible to infections from local injuries, which results in more scarring and additional lymphedema. Infections of the limbs, called cellulitis, often develop after even minor cuts or abrasions and they can only be controlled with long-term antibiotics.

You can assist your patient following a procedure which puts him at risk for lymphedema by encouraging good nutrition with a high protein diet and active physical exercise to help the muscles pump the lymphatic fluid. It is important for him to control his weight, as obesity only increases the risk of lymphedema. No matter how much effort you and your patient put into a prevention program, however, lymphedema may occur, either immediately after surgery, or it may occur years later. The most important factor in preventing and controlling lymphedema is the exercising of muscles. Walking or bicycling can improve lymphatic flow. Breast cancer patients are usually instructed to go through a series of hand and arm exercises after surgery. A similar program might be prescribed for patients with any of the cancers involving limbs. You might assist your patient in the prevention and control of lymphedema by encouraging him to do all or some of the following:

- elevate the affected limb whenever possible
- clean and lubricate the skin daily
- use extra caution to prevent injury or infection
- use an electric razor
- avoid walking barefoot
- wear gloves while gardening or doing household chores
- minimize invasive procedures such as drawing blood
- take good care of nails and cuticles
- avoid extreme hot or cold on affected swollen limb
- while sitting, change position every thirty minutes
- faithfully exercise
- watch for signs of infection

Encourage your patient to continue to practice protective procedures as a routine since lymphedema can come back at any time if an injury occurs.

• Sleep Problems: Sleep problems often accompany serious illness because of pain, anxiety, worry, or night sweats. Sleep problems may include the inability to sleep as much as needed or sleeping more than usual. Any changes in usual sleep habits can be defined as sleep problems. Most often these are temporary and can be dealt with by pure common sense. As a caregiver, you can play a significant role in assisting your patient to have more comfortable nights. This will result in more comfortable nights for you as well.

Sleeping more than usual is to be expected. Fighting a serious illness takes a lot of energy. Frequent naps and sleeping eight or more hours a night is completely acceptable. But more often, the inability to sleep is the problem. You can help your patient get enough sleep by:

- keeping his sheets clean and neatly tucked in and free from wrinkles
- making sure his sleep environment is quiet, attractive and comfortable
- establishing schedules for naps and bedtime
- offering decaffeinated beverages or a back rub before bedtime.

If medication has been prescribed for your patient to assist with sleep, make sure that he takes it as directed and be aware that the use of this medication should be considered temporary.

There are many other possible side effects that might be experienced by your patient, including frequent falling, blood clots, radiation burns, fevers, infections, and sexual problems. Find out what you are most likely to deal with early in the process. Learning how to make your patient more comfortable while getting through these unpleasant side effects will make you feel more successful as a caregiver.

Why, I Felt Like Tammy Faye Baker!

My friend, Terry, recently completed treatment for breast cancer including chemotherapy. She sent me the following note via E-mail, making me smile for the rest of the day.

"I was so excited today! It seems when eyelashes start to grow back all of a sudden, they're back! I lifted my lid this morning and lo and behold there was a whole row of eyelashes! I grabbed my eyelash curler and curled those babies and put on layer after layer of mascara to make up for the past seven months! Why, I felt like Tammy Faye Baker! Little things like this can make me so happy!"

NOTES

To better understand the disease, treatment and possible side effects, I need to:

Stop by the library for:

_____
_____
_____
_____
_____
_____
_____
_____
_____

Look up_____

On the Internet.

Call:

_____
_____
_____
_____
_____
_____
_____
_____
_____

Chapter 7

Emotional Issues

You gain strength, courage and confidence by every
experience in which you really stop to look fear in the face.

Eleanor Roosevelt

As caregivers we experience a range of emotions we might not have experienced before we found ourselves in this role. Fear is the word spoken most often by caregivers. Knowledge can help reduce the fear of the unknown and help us be realistic about the future. Talking with someone about our fears helps us to think through the reasons for our feelings. We might experience a sense of loss or sorrow for what a person used to be and may never again be. We may feel sad about how the direction of our own lives has taken a turn due to this illness. Oddly, guilt is another feeling we experience more often than most people might imagine. We feel guilty because we think we should have recognized sooner that the person was ill. Or, we are well and the person we love is sick. Or, we are older and a younger sibling or friend shouldn't have to suffer. We might feel guilty for being mad at the patient because he was a smoker and brought on his own illness. The best way for us to handle this guilt is to discuss it openly with the patient and forgive each other. If we do not, we waste precious time and energy that could be put to better use.

Talking openly with a seriously ill person can be very difficult. Sometimes a patient does not want to talk at all and our job is to be available if he does. On the other hand, we may hear words we don't really want to hear. When this occurs, we must remember we do not have to resolve all issues; only that we need to listen.

When we find ourselves disagreeing with our patients about such things as the choice of treatment, we must understand how important it is for the patient to retain some control over his life. Even if we are sure something would be better, we need to recognize that our job is to support. One of the best ways we can provide this support is by working with a health care professional on behalf of the patient. Researching treatment options or resolving insurance issues can be an exhausting experience. Handling the business side of an illness can relieve a great amount of stress and allow the patient to focus on decisions about his treatment.

Anger, fear and self-esteem are three emotions that need a great deal of attention. These emotions are felt by both the patient and the caregiver and need to be resolved so that depression and resignation don't take over. Being angry saps you both of energy that can be channeled into coping with disease and living life with as much quality as possible. Help your patient to identify his anger and express it. Do whatever is required to work it out, short of hurting someone else. Let your patient hit pillows, scream or cry. But get him to talk about why he is angry. Fear can be a terrible master and working through that fear can literally save your life and your patient's life. If both you and your patient fully understand the ramifications of the patient's disease as well as what to expect during treatment, fear can be resolved. It is important to allow others to express their fears to you as a caregiver, even to the patient. Share with them your knowledge of the disease and treatment to help put them at ease as well. Self-esteem can be greatly affected by the very idea of having a disease or having a loved one with a disease. It is common to feel that being a better person might have prevented this from happening, as though it is some sort of divine punishment. Reassure your patient that this is a superstitious belief and believe it yourself.

Regardless of prognosis, coping with a serious illness and treatment of a loved one can be time-consuming and energy sapping. Negative emotions will consume every waking moment if you allow them to do so. By doing your best to not give up hope and maintaining a positive attitude, both you and your patient will benefit in the months ahead, making the entire process easier to bear.

I Never Had the Chance...

My brother was diagnosed with a malignant brain tumor only ten short days before his death. The ten days were spent in the hospital – hearing the diagnosis, authorizing a biopsy, and fearing what would happen next. Before we could arrange what was next, it was over. I never had the opportunity to sit with him and talk about what was important to him or to me while we were growing up. I didn't get to help with physical therapy or plan meals. I didn't have time to accept what was happening or ask what he wanted done after his death. It was all up to my mother, my two sisters and me to make a lot of decisions that should have been made by my brother. It took a very long time to deal with his death. Now I understand that if we had been able to participate in his illness for some time, it might have made his death easier for him and for us, the survivors.

Making Us All More Comfortable

Late one September, my mother went into diabetic shock and called the paramedics. Two days after she was admitted to the hospital, we were informed she had pancreatic cancer. It had already spread to her liver. The doctor estimated 2-3 months of life for her, but she died in 5 weeks. There were three of us, my sisters and I, and we each spent part of every day or evening with her. We did what we could to make her more comfortable. There were days it seemed she would get well. Other days, she could barely speak. We did so many things that were futile, but it kept us busy and we wanted to believe it made her more comfortable. We were also trying to make us more comfortable. I remember that she loved the music of John Tesh, so I took a portable tape player and some tapes for her. I don't think she heard any of them. We put photos of her children and grandchildren on the walls of her room. We talked and we laughed and we cried. For the last week or so, we talked to her and touched her and watched as each breath became slower and slower, until, at last, there was no life left to breathe.

Parents Are Not Supposed to Bury Their Children

When my brother was diagnosed with a malignant brain tumor at the age of 45, my mother repeatedly said, "Mothers are not supposed to bury their children." She was broken hearted when he died ten days later and she never got over it. Many parents are faced with losing children at all ages. The fact that my brother was 45 years old made him no less of a child to my mother. When my friend died at age 51 of pancreatic cancer, her mother cried no less than if she had been 5, 15 or 25.

When Don's young son, 19 years old, suddenly broke a leg while getting out of his small truck, it was determined he had bone cancer. He had the leg amputated and lived for about two more years, the cancer eventually taking him. The parents never gave up hope, but have lived with the pain of his death ever since. Don, like so many other parents, will never understand why it happened to his child.

We Laugh, We Cry

At 3:00 a.m., my husband stirred and I jumped out of bed, offering pain medication or sleeping pills to put him at ease. I checked his catheter and when he was settled I tiptoed to the guestroom where my sister was gently turning over to minimize her own pain. "Can I get you a Vicodin?" I whispered, trying not to startle her. "I'm not taking Vicodin," she reminded me, "I'm taking Darvon." I laughed and said,

"Want one anyway?" She laughed too, ever so carefully as each move hurt. I got her the Darvon she needed. She thanked me and I hugged her. I walked slowly up the stairs, sat down on the floor near the windows in the moonlight and cried for both of them and for the unfairness of the separate cancer battles they were fighting.

NOTES

I'll make every effort to:

- Encourage open discussion
- Talk about my own issues
- Think of something positive at least once a day
- Smile often

Chapter 8

Spiritual Issues

Your faith is what you believe, not what you know.

John Lancaster Spalding

Caregivers, like patients, worry about spiritual issues. Working with one who is very ill or dying can bring up very difficult issues for us. Perhaps we are feeling the unfairness of the situation, fear about what will really happen to the person when they die, or fear about our own deaths. Having these doubts makes it more difficult to be of assistance to our patients when they want to discuss their concerns. For those patients whose faith gives answers and comfort, our support of that faith will be both helpful and appreciated. For those troubled by uncertainty, we can help by sharing our own uncertainties, showing that their concerns are normal. If the patient is receptive to such an idea, a member of the clergy might be invited to meet with the patient. Let the person for whom you are caring know you will be happy to arrange visits, but do not force it. Remember that your views may be quite different than the patient's, and you must be careful to accept and respect his views. Encourage and support him in his faith. Offer to provide tapes of hymns or religious music they might enjoy. A religious symbol such as a Bible or a rosary might be comforting.

Religion is a source of strength for many of us. Others have never had strong religious beliefs and feel no desire to turn to religion at such a time. Always let the patient be your guide and never impose.

Don't Take My Sister

By the time I realized that I was shouting in the hospital chapel, a friendly arm was around my shoulder. I had visited this chapel more than once in the two months since my sister had been diagnosed with colon cancer. This time was very different. Linda was in the emergency room with a chest full of blood clots. My husband was scheduled for his own cancer surgery the next day. My other sister was going through radiation treatments for yet another form of cancer. Only six months before, my mother lost her battle with pancreatic cancer. "Enough is enough!" I screamed at the empty altar. "Stop hurting the people I love. All this talk about God not giving you more than you can handle…well, I'm here to tell you I have as much as I can handle. Please don't take my sister from me." I had reached the point of pain and fear for my family that I was overwhelmed. The friendly arm, I believe, belonged to one of the nuns at the hospital. She did not preach. She did not remind me to put my faith in God. She just put her arms around me and held me until my sobs changed to whimpers. Then she quietly left me alone in the chapel. I do not regularly attend church, but I have returned to that chapel many times since that day to give thanks that my sister is still with me.

Whatever, Lord

When Maria, a pretty brunette of about 35 came to the resource library, she was about to begin six months of chemotherapy for Hodgkin's Disease. She was calm and eager to learn what she could do to help herself get through it with the least amount of impact to her life and her family. I was impressed with her approach to the research and, in the hour we spent together, I began to understand her calmness. She referred to her situation as "part of the journey" and commented to her sister how fortunate it was for her that a particular doctor was available to take her as a patient. She followed this statement by a simple, "thank you, God." As she was leaving, I asked if she was aware that the hospital boutique offered wigs, hats and the like. She was and had scheduled an appointment the next day for a wig fitting. She said she just couldn't imagine herself bald. I commented that sometimes hair color and texture change after chemotherapy and perhaps in six months she would be a blond. She chuckled as she left, looked toward the heavens and said, "Whatever, Lord!"

A Big Surprise

Some things are never quite explained. I have a cherished memory of my mother that I can't begin to explain. Because my sister shared this event, I know that I did not imagine it. It's one of those things that I just keep tucked away and it makes me smile from time to time.

My mother had been diagnosed with pancreatic cancer and it was suggested that we put her in a nursing home until such time that she might be strong enough to go home. We wanted her to be as comfortable as possible in her new surroundings. A few days after Mother was admitted, she felt strong enough to have her hair washed. So we took her to the salon in the home and then for a tour so she could see more of her new environment.

We went out into the large lobby where patients gathered with families and friends for visits. It was a cheerful room with lots of windows allowing sunlight to filter through. We settled in for a visit: Mom in her wheelchair and the two of us on a sofa. Mother spotted a piano in the corner and asked that we push her over to it. We did and she moved from her wheelchair to the piano bench and began to play. My sister, having gone around to the other side of the piano to take a picture, thought that I was playing a trick on her and that it was a player piano! I was as shocked as my sister was. We had never heard our mother play the piano. She played a familiar tune that brought other visitors to the room. I remember the smile on her face, as though she had really pulled something on us. When we questioned her about when she had learned to play the piano, she simply said that she had always wanted to play. She died a few weeks later and we never did learn the source of her spontaneous performance, but we think we know.

I Don't Think I'm Finished Here

Georgia was married to a minister, Tom, and she was the mother of his four children. When he was diagnosed with pancreatic cancer, he began the usual treatments and understood the seriousness of the disease. When the traditional treatments had been exhausted, they began pursuing alternative medicines and procedures in an attempt to keep him from losing his fight with the disease. They prayed together and they truly believed that God's message to them indicated that Tom's work was not yet finished. They, therefore, did not seriously consider the possibility that Tom would soon die. People diagnosed with grave illnesses often go through periods of denial and simply refuse to accept what fate has in store for them. Having spent an evening with Georgia, I truly do not believe either she or Tom was in denial in that sense. I don't believe I have ever met a person with such an unshakable faith. It was not that she was denying the disease, but simply that she believed God was communicating with them and she trusted Him. My heart was warmed by her faith and yet I felt sad for her because she did not prepare herself or her children for Tom's death.

NOTES
I'll offer to discuss spiritual issues but not push.
I'll be true to my own spiritual beliefs.
I'll respect my patient's choices.

Chapter 9

Hostile Patient / Hostile Caregiver

When the rock is hard, we get harder than the rock.
When the job is tough, we get tougher than the job.

George Cullum, Sr.

Patients with serious illnesses are oftentimes angry about being sick and will direct this anger at their caregivers because it is "safe". They can be belligerent, demanding, or downright mean. This type of patient is not likely to have much compassion for the efforts of their caregiver. You can deal with this best by getting some help.

A friend, an oncology nurse, once told me that cancer doesn't make people nicer. She said that if someone is already ill tempered by nature, he isn't going to be any nicer just because he knows he's dying, he'll probably be worse. It certainly makes the task of caring for the patient more difficult. This is the time when the caregiver needs a lot of support from others. This isn't easy because the patient is often quite vocal about who he will allow to bathe him, feed him, and bring him his medications. It is important for caregivers to plan time for themselves during these difficult periods.

Even if the patient objects, suggest trying additional help for short periods of time or for certain tasks. Be realistic about what to expect from the patient. Don't expect perfection out of yourself, even if the patient does! Being a caregiver is a difficult task and everyone makes mistakes.

Anger is most often the response to the fears and frustrations that are a normal part of the journey through a serious illness. Most patients and some caregivers do their best to ignore these emotions. But they don't go away, and often instead produce anger as a cover-up. As a caregiver, it is imperative that you be sensitive to why the anger is there and give your patient permission to be angry. This is not the same as allowing him to be abusive, but rather allowing him to experience and deal with the emotion. Once you have done this, you can begin to talk more openly. By moving from this place of anger, you will both be better equipped to deal with the real issues you are facing.

Why Am I Yelling at You?

Caregivers, like patients, can become hostile. Hostility stems from the anger you might feel for any number of reasons. The patient might be demanding or irritating at times. Friends and family might not be as helpful as you would like them to be. Or you may blame the patient for getting sick, such as the smoker who contracts lung cancer.

It is quite normal to get angry. Your world has suddenly turned chaotic and uncertain by the illness of a loved one. Here are a few tips that may help when you're feeling angry.

- Express anger before it gets too severe
- Make an extra effort to understand the other person's point of view
- Get away from the situation for awhile, even a few hours
- Talk with someone who doesn't tend to be judgmental.

In Sickness and in Health

After Larry had back surgery, he was recovering in a hospital bed in the living room of the small apartment he shared with his wife, Sharon. He was in considerable pain for weeks and bedridden for months. They were in their early twenties and had been married only two years.

Sharon was working full time 20 miles from home. Larry demanded his sheets be changed daily, even though they had no washer or dryer. He wanted specific meals at certain times. He complained each day about the water for his bed bath being too hot or too cold. Sharon went home during her lunch break each day to make his lunch and change the channel on the television. Larry was truly an unpleasant patient and Sharon shed many tears at the laundromat while washing his sheets. A few years later, he dumped her. It happens.

What Will I Do When You're Gone?

"You are dying and I need some help here. I don't know what to do." Shirley regretted those words, spoken to her husband, the minute she said them. Actually, she regrets them to this day. Caregivers, like patients, experience fear and frustration. Shirley's husband owned his own business and hadn't shared any financial details with Shirley during their years of marriage and certainly not since his cancer diagnosis. She was so afraid of losing him and of not knowing what should be done about the business upon his death. He, on the other hand, did not want to discuss anything. Perhaps to him it meant accepting his fate or giving up. If he had helped her through this, his death would have been no less traumatic. However, the months of frustration and red tape that followed might have been lessened. He left her with no choice but to deal with all of the financial problems one-by-one.

Just a Couple of Puppies

Ruth has cared for her husband, Jim, for the ten years in which he has been battling two different types of cancer. He survived colon cancer, only to be faced with an attack to his nasal passages, resulting in severe surgery and radiation. His sinuses, palate and entire mouth area have been affected. He cannot eat any solid food and must wear a prosthesis in his mouth to prevent his liquid meals from backing up into his nasal passages. Jim misses the taste of food and the joy of sharing a meal with others. He has become bitter and refuses to go to restaurants, even on Ruth's birthday to join the celebration.

Ruth has accepted her role as primary caregiver but confided to me that it sometimes hurts that Jim does not try to reciprocate for all of the care and attention that is showered on him. Recently, her neighbors found that they must move and cannot take their two beagles with them. Ruth has cared for these dogs while her neighbors have been on vacation and has bonded with them. The neighbors have offered the dogs to her. Jim says, absolutely not. It has nothing to do with health reasons. He says they will tear up the lawn and that she feeds the dogs before she feeds him! He has gone as far as to say that if she wants the dogs, she can move out! How sad that Jim cannot see the pleasure the dogs would bring to Ruth, and possibly to him as well. So Ruth has joined a group that gathers on weekends to walk their dogs in a park. She just joins in, without a dog, and enjoys the animals that others bring. Jim has no idea how lucky he is to have Ruth.

NOTES

In the event of anger, I'll encourage discussion and express my own feelings.

I will not tolerate abuse.

I will not be abusive.

Chapter 10

Getting Help from Others

We expect more of ourselves than we have any right to.

Oliver Wendell Holmes, Jr.

When illness strikes a family, loved ones tend to assume particular roles. Some deal well with the illness and provide continuous support. Others are unable to cope with the possibility of death and completely disappear. Some simply say they are uncomfortable around sick people. Those of us who assume the responsibilities of caregiving must understand that everyone handles serious illness in a different way and recognizing this, we can gain assistance from some of those who might otherwise shy away. If friends or family don't call, call them. They may simply be unsure of what is needed. Ask for assistance with small things such as picking up a prescription, preparing a meal or stopping by for a short visit. This will often bring others into the circle and make them comfortable enough to continue to provide you with support. Most people are very happy to have something suggested to them that they can do to help. Assistance with shopping or transportation to a doctor's appointment can be a huge help to the patient and the caregiver.

While it hardly seems fair that the primary caregiver has to take responsibility for directing the efforts of others when we are having difficulty just keeping our own lives going, the rewards can make the effort well worth it. Once family members and friends are no longer reluctant to help, they will do many things on their own. True friends will stick with you throughout the process and be there for you when you need help the most. The help might be in the form of a casserole for dinner or a warm and caring hug. It might be in the form of an afternoon visit, assistance with completing insurance forms or long-stemmed roses. Everyone has something to offer at times like this. If there is a family member who loves to shop, she might be asked to assist with Christmas shopping. Perhaps a cousin will offer to do a shampoo or a manicure. Someone might offer to write notes acknowledging cards, flowers and gifts. Day-to-day chores don't go away. Let a neighbor dust or vacuum if they offer. Keeping a list of tasks that need to be done can be helpful when offers for help arrive.

I once heard someone say, "Winners are people who spend time doing the things losers are uncomfortable doing." Caregivers are winners. YOU are a winner.

When a patient reaches the final phase of a terminal illness, additional help is available that will enable him to live an alert, pain-free life and to manage other symptoms so that his last days may be spent with dignity and quality at home or in a home-like setting. Hospice care is available to terminally ill patients who no longer wish treatment to cure their disease and who have a limited life expectancy (6 months or less). A doctor, family members, friends, clergy or health professionals may refer patients to Hospice. Hospice is a coordinated program of supportive service and symptom control for terminally ill patients and their families. Hospice is primarily a concept of care, not a specific place of care. Hospice services may be provided to patients at home, or in a skilled nursing facility. Hospice offers palliative, rather than curative treatment. Under the direction of a physician, Hospice uses sophisticated methods of pain and symptom management that enables the patient to live as fully and comfortably as possible. Hospice treats the person, not the disease utilizing a team made up of professionals who address the medical, emotional, psychological and spiritual needs of the patient. Emphasis is placed on the quality, rather than the length of life. Hospice neither hastens nor postpones death. It affirms life and regards death as a normal process. This support is offered on a 24-hour a day, seven days a week basis. Assistance is also available with financial planning, assessing family needs, and assisting with funeral arrangements. After the patient dies, bereavement counseling by the Hospice team assists the family to continue living as fully as possible.

All too often, the doctor and perhaps the family, waits until death is only weeks or days away before asking for assistance from Hospice. Getting this support earlier in the process can be of great benefit to the patient and to the family by helping everyone involved to understand the near death and death experience. This help is only a phone call away.

We Never Know

Donna was a former employee who became a friend. She worked for me when my mother was diagnosed with pancreatic cancer. I shared many details with her during that time and grew close to her because she cared enough to ask every day and really listened when I told her about my mother's illness. A year later Donna was diagnosed with pancreatic cancer. She was terrified, but told me that because I had been so open with her she knew what to expect and would have been afraid to ask for herself. During the next year, I saw Donna in the hospital and at home and became acquainted with her family. I offered what comfort I could, crying all the way home from each visit. She was lucky to have a close and supportive family and I was lucky to see them together. She died at home with Hospice assisting the family. I still keep in touch with her mother and feel that my life is richer for having gotten to know this woman, even in death.

NOTES
I will keep a list of tasks that need to be done.
I will never refuse help from anyone who offers.
I will ask for help when I need it.

Chapter 11

Taking Care of Yourself

If a man would move the world, he must first move himself.

Socrates

Once we accept the task of becoming a caregiver, we must recognize the importance of taking good care of ourselves. We will be of no use to anyone if our own physical and emotional health becomes impaired during the course of our caregiving duties. Although this task is not an easy one, there is comfort in the knowledge that we are needed. The better we perform this task, the more confidence we have in our ability to care for and give dignity to those who need our help.

No matter how overwhelming the experience may be, it cannot be stressed enough how important it is to make sure we have some time for ourselves each week, and preferably each day. This isn't always possible, but striving toward this goal will ensure some time is saved for us. At least once a week we should plan a lunch with a friend, see a movie, or play tennis. It may seem selfish, but this diversion will make us less stressed and better caregivers.

Caregivers frequently do not eat properly. Some overeat and others don't eat enough. Just as we are concerned our patients get the right balance of nutrition each day; we should be concerned for ourselves. Using food as comfort can lead to weight gain. Eating on the run can become a bad habit. When others ask what they can do to help, ask them to prepare a meal and drop by with it. If the patient is not eating well because he cannot tolerate food, we must remember to continue fueling our bodies to be most effective as caregivers.

Exercise too, plays an important role in maintaining our health. It is not practical to suggest an hour or two a day at a gym during this time. But a 30-minute walk or an exercise video that keeps us in the next room can lower our risk of becoming ill. Finding a physical activity that we enjoy will also make us more mentally alert.

Although easier said than done, we know it is important that we make every effort to get a good night's rest. The number of hours of sleep we require is different for each individual. Know that number for your patient. Patients may not sleep well during treatment due to pain, anxiety, night sweats or any number of side effects resulting from their illnesses. We may not sleep because our patients don't or, due to our own despair or sadness. Sleeping well is very important to the healing process and every effort should be made to make the patient comfortable at bedtime. Avoid stimulants late in the day, and maintain a schedule as much as possible. There will be times this is difficult due to chemotherapy or radiation treatments that might render the patient extremely tired and temporarily requiring several naps a day.

As caregivers, we must learn to accept help from others. We must not be afraid to ask for help and we should never decline an offer of help from anyone. If a neighbor offers to grocery shop, or come in and sit with the patient for an hour or so, graciously accept. Be prepared with an answer to the question, "What can I do to help?"

As we commit ourselves to being caregivers, we must also commit to taking the best possible care of our fellow caregivers and ourselves. We all need the comfort and encouragement that can only come from within this circle of those who have chosen to excel as caregivers.

NOTES

These are the things I miss most since becoming a caregiver:

_____

_____

_____

_____

_____

_____

_____

_____

_____

_____

I will include at least one of these things in my life each week.
I will take a few minutes each day to do something just for me.
I will reach out to other caregivers.

Chapter 12

Support Groups

Down in their hearts, wise men know this truth: the only way to help yourself is to help others.

Elbert Hubbard

Support groups aren't for everyone. Over the past few years, more and more types of support groups have become available to caregivers as well as patients. The quality and type of support groups available vary but most have the goal of providing a place where caregivers can learn technical skills, share experiences and gain emotional support from each other. You may have to try a couple of different groups until you find the one that best meets your needs. This may be a group that is for both the patient and the caregiver. Usually in this group, the patients and caregivers are divided for some portion of the meeting to allow each to speak freely without the other present. Other groups are for caregivers only. If you are the type of individual who is willing to share experiences and learn from those of others, you might want to consider the following points when selecting a support group.

Is the group for the specific type of caregiving you are doing? A group specific to cancer or Alzheimer's, for example, will put you in with others dealing with the same situations.

Are the group leaders trained in facilitating such groups? Leadership skills can make the difference between a successful group and a negative one.

Has the leader been a caregiver? Personal experience can be very valuable and garners empathy.

Has the group been around for awhile? Good groups last while others fade quickly.

Does the meeting schedule suit your schedule? Once you get involved and find the group helpful, you will find that you will make the time to attend.

Once you have decided that you'd like to participate in a support group and know essentially what type, you can find out what is offered in your area through your doctor's office or local hospital. You might also find this information through organizations that are involved with your particular needs, such as the Alzheimer's Association. The Internet offers on-line caregiver support groups. While some caregivers find these groups somewhat impersonal, others prefer them because they can remain anonymous and don't have to leave home to attend.

Many caregivers are reluctant to attend support groups because they don't want to become emotional in front of strangers. In many cases, these strangers quickly become friends because they have such a common bond. Everyone has their turn to laugh and to cry and a group who truly understands the challenges they face surrounds them. Taking the time to attend support groups can provide us with a source of physical and emotional support that is hard to find elsewhere. It is also another way to take care of ourselves while enhancing our caregiving skills.

NOTES

I'll consider joining a support group in my area. They are:

_____

_____

_____

_____

_____

_____

_____

_____

Or visit a support group on-line:

_____

_____

_____

_____

_____

_____

_____

Or talk with at least one other caregiver to gain and offer support:

_____

_____

_____

_____

_____

_____

Chapter 13

Moving on

*Worry is a thin stream of fear trickling through the mind.
If encouraged, it cuts a channel into which all other
thoughts are drained.*

Arthur Somers Roche

Anyone whose life has been affected by his own serious illness or that of a loved one will not forget it. We move on, but we are constantly alert to signs like colds or headaches or sweats that might be cause for panic. Caregivers, like patients, feel this forever. While the illness may have robbed us of the illusion that once led us to believe our days on earth were limitless, we are now extremely aware that each day is a precious gift. Our loved ones may be living with artificial limbs, breast changes, or fatigue. Or they may no longer be with us. We have taken a good look at our own lives and have decided what is really important to us. Perhaps we have become more assertive and more compassionate as a result of our experiences. We have new attitudes toward work and play and relationships. We have begun to eliminate frivolous people and superficial activities from our lives because we want every moment to count.

Fear of recurrence is common to survivors of serious illnesses and for their caregivers. You can help your patient and yourself minimize this fear by maintaining an optimistic attitude, being vigilant about regular checkups, and leading a healthy lifestyle. Eating a balanced diet, exercising regularly, and not smoking will help you both live your lives to the fullest.

We hope and pray we will never again sit by the bedside of a dying loved one, but we know we have the courage and strength to do it if we must.

"Are You Going to Heaven, Too?"

Todd was going to the doctor for a routine checkup for a back problem and had his four-year son, Michael, with him. When they arrived at the medical complex, Todd helped Michael out of the car and noticed that his eyes were filled with tears. Todd asked what was wrong. "Are you going to heaven, too?" Michael asked. Todd suddenly realized that his young son remembered this medical facility from the many visits there when his mother was dying of breast cancer. She had died just months before.

It was at this point that Todd understood for the first time just how much a small child understands and retains. From that point on, Todd knew he had to choose his words very carefully. He helped Michael to understand his mommy had been very sick and his daddy's back just hurt. He explained that the doctor would fix the hurt. Now Todd must be cautious when referring to the children or anyone they love as being sick, even with the flu, in order to keep Michael from worrying that everyone who is sick will soon be going to heaven.

First We Keep You Alive

When my husband was diagnosed with prostate cancer, our biggest fear was that the cancer had spread to other parts of his body. Having determined there was no metastasis, I began to deal with an entirely different set of rules for the caregiver. We got through the surgery, the catheter experience, the regaining of strength. Now we know he will live. He has regained continence and his quality of life has returned to almost normal…almost. Sexuality is now an issue. During diagnosis and treatment, this didn't seem so important because life and death discussions took precedence. But now, months later, he is alive, he is dry and he is frustrated because he has lost a part of his manhood. Here is yet another kind of "caregiving" that goes on every day. No, I don't have to feed and bathe him or provide him medical care. But I do have to reassure him he is still loved and comfort him and be there and it isn't always easy because he is angry and sad and wants life to be what it was before…and so do I.

NOTES
My new attitudes:

_____

_____

_____

_____

_____

_____

_____

_____

_____

_____

_____

_____

What I'm doing to maximize an optimistic attitude for the future:

_____

_____

_____

_____

_____

_____

_____

_____

_____

_____

_____

_____

Chapter 14

Final Thoughts

*Those who bring sunshine to the lives of others
cannot keep it from them.*

Sir James M. Barrie

I have written this book because I have talked with dozens of people whose lives have been seriously impacted by the illness or death of a loved one. Each has a story to tell. Some stories are beautiful, even if they don't end the way we would have liked. Others are very sad not only because of the illness but because a few simple guidelines for the patient and the caregiver might have made the process more gentle.

While I have had some involvement as a caregiver to a mother, brother, two sisters, and a husband – all cancer patients, I was blessed because each one was loving and caring, and appreciative of the slightest effort on my part. I know they understood throughout the process that when they hurt, I hurt. I offer my heartfelt thanks to my husband, Bruce, and my sisters, JoAnne and Linda for helping me help them. It is my hope that sharing these experiences and some practical advice will benefit others who are feeling the pain of a suffering loved one.

I Look in the Mirror

I look in the mirror, at this tired face,
An unspoken record of events taken place,
Dark circles, deep lines clearly show the fear,
That has been so much a part of this past year.
There has been so much illness – a sister, a friend.

I constantly ask, when will it end?
I give thanks for every WELL day, treasured as never before,
And pray for a cure, nothing less, nothing more.

Each has shown courage, rarely a complaint or a tear,
I wonder if they realize my incredible fear.
A New Year approaches, the deep lines remain,
A reminder forever, of the sadness and pain.

A New Year approaches, a renewed faith is in place,
As I look in the mirror, at this tired face.

Karen L. Twichell

NOTES

I'll remember to reach out to caregivers in the future, when I have more time, and share what the experience has taught me.

Caregivers I'll call:

_____

_____

_____

_____

_____

_____

_____

_____

_____

_____

About the Author

Karen L. Twichell was first introduced to the world of caregiving when her grandmother was diagnosed with cancer twenty-five years ago. Since then, her mother, father and brother have all lost their battles with cancer. She has two sisters and a husband who are cancer survivors. Diabetes and heart disease have also impacted her family. After a thirty-year corporate management career, she has written this book in an attempt to help other caregivers cope with the task that many face and no one wants.

Karen lives in Newport Beach, California, is a public speaker on caregiving, facilitates a support group for cancer survivors and their caregivers and hosts a chat room for caregivers on the Internet.

Karen may be contacted at kltwichell@aol.com

Resource Listing

A

AIDS Clinical Trials
Information Service
P. O. Box 6421
Rockville, MD 20849-6421   Telephone 800-874-2572

Alzheimer's Association
919 N. Michigan Avenue, Suite 1000
Chicago, IL 60611   Telephone 312-335-8700

Alzheimer's Disease Education & Referral Center
P. O. Box 8250
Silver Spring, MD 20907-8250   Telephone 301-495-3311

Alzheimer's Family Care
12051 Indian Creek Court
Beltsville, MD 20705   Telephone 800-777-3264

American Association of Homes & Services for the Aging
AAHSA Publications
Department 5119
Washington, DC 20061-5119   Telephone 800-508-9442

American Association of Retired Persons (AARP)
601 "E" Street, NW
Washington, DC 20049   Telephone 800-434-3410

American Bar Association
Commission on Legal Problems of the Elderly
740 15th Street, NW, 8th Floor
Washington, DC 20005   Telephone 202-662-8690

American Cancer Society
1599 Clifton Road, NE
Atlanta, GA 30329   Telephone 800-227-2345

American Foundation for Urological Disease, Inc.
300 West Pratt Street, Suite 401
Baltimore, MD 21201   Telephone 410-727-2908

American Heart Association
7272 Greenville Avenue
Dallas, TX 75231-4596   Telephone 800-553-6321

American Kidney Fund
6110 Executive Boulevard, Suite 100
Rockville, MD 20852   Telephone 800-638-8299

American Parkinson Disease Association
1250 Hylan Boulevard, Suite 4B
Staten Island, NY 10305   Telephone 800-223-2732

American Self-Help Clearinghouse
(Information Clearinghouse for Caregivers and other Groups)
25 Pocono Road
Denville, NJ 07834-2995   Telephone 201-625-7101

B
Bone Marrow Transplant
Family Support Network, Inc.
P. O. Box 845
Avon, CT 06001   Telephone 800-826-9376

C
Cancer Care, Inc.
1180 Avenue of the Americas
New York, NY 10036   Telephone 212-302-2400

Cancervive
6500 Wilshire Boulevard, Suite 500
Los Angeles, CA 90048   Telephone 310-203-9232

Candlelighters Childhood Cancer Foundation
7910 Woodmont Avenue, Suite 460
Bethesda, MD 20814-3015   Telephone 800-366-2223

CDC National AIDS Hotline
P. O. Box 13827
Research Triangle Park, NC 27709   Telephone 800-342-2437

Children of Aging Parents (CAPS)
1609 Woodburn Road, Suite 302A
Levittown, PA 19055   Telephone 800-227-7294

Children of Parkinsonians (COPS)
73-700 El Paseo, Suite 2
Palm Desert, CA 92260   Telephone 760-773-5628

Cooperative Caring Network
(Sponsored by United Seniors Health Cooperative)
1331 "H" Street, NW, Suite 500
Washington, DC 20005   Telephone 202-393-7736

Council of Better Business Bureaus, Inc.
Publications Department
4200 Wilson Boulevard, Suite 800
Arlington, VA 22203   Telephone 703-276-0100

D
Department of Veteran Affairs
Geriatric and Extended Care Health Group
810 Vermont Avenue, NW
Washington, DC 20420   Telephone 202-273-8540

Directory of Adult Respite
Care Funded or Provided by State Governments
919 N. Michigan Avenue, Suite 100
Chicago, IL 60611   Telephone 800-272-3900

Double Check
(Locates services for caregivers of the elderly)
P. O. Box 1963
Springfield, OH 45501-1963   Telephone 800-480-4359

E
Elder Support Network
(Service of Association of Jewish Family & Children's Agencies)
3086 Highway 27, Suite 1
P. O. Box 248
Kendall Park, NJ 08824   Telephone 800-634-7346

Eldercare Locator
National Association of Area Agencies on Aging
1112 16th Street, NW, Suite 100
Washington, DC 20036　　　　　　Telephone 800-677-1116

F
Family Caregiver Alliance
425 Bush Street, Suite 500
San Francisco, CA 94108　　　　　Telephone 800-445-8106

Family Friends Resource Center
National Council on Aging
Director of Intergenerational Programs
409 Third Street, SW, 2nd Floor
Washington, DC 20024　　　　　　Telephone 202-479-6675

Federal Hill-Burton Free Care Program
5600 Fishers Lane
Park Lawn Boulevard #7-47
Rockville, MD 20857　　　　　　　Telephone 800-638-0742

Federal National Mortgage Association (FANNIEMAE)
Public Information Office
3900 Wisconsin Avenue, NW
Washington, DC 20016　　　　　　Telephone 800-732-6643

G

H

I

Institute of Certified Financial Planners
3801 E. Florida Avenue, Suite 708
Denver, CO 80210   Telephone 800-282-7526

International Association for Financial Planning
5775 Glenridge Drive, NE, Suite B300
Atlanta, GA 30328-5364   Telephone 800-945-4237

J

K

KAIROS
AIDS Caregiving Organization
2128 15th Street
San Francisco, CA 94114   Telephone 415-861-0877

Kent Waldrep National Paralysis Foundation
16415 Addison Road, Suite 550
Dallas, TX 75248   Telephone 800-925-2873

L

M

Man to Man
(Network for caregivers and loved ones with prostate cancer)
910 Contento Street
Sarasota, FL 34242   Telephone 941-349-1719

March of Dimes Birth Defects Foundation
National Office

1275 Mamaroneck Avenue
White Plains, NY 10605   Telephone 914 428 7100

Medicare Consumer Line
P. O. Box 5798
Timonium, MD 21094-5298   Telephone 410-771-8080
                                     Telephone 410-252-5310

(The) Mended Hearts, Inc.
(Support for Heart Disease Patients and Family)
7272 Greenville Avenue
Dallas, TX 75231-4596   Telephone 214-706-1442

Multiple Sclerosis Foundation
6350 N. Andrews Avenue
Fort Lauderdale, FL 33309   Telephone 800-441-7055

MUMS
National Parent-to-Parent Network
150 Custer Court
Green Bay, WI 54301-5333   Telephone 414-336-5333

N
National Academy of Elder Law Attorneys (NAELA)
1604 North Country Club Road
Tucson, AZ 85716   Telephone 520-881-4005

National Adult Day Services Associations
National Council on Aging
409 3rd Street SW, Suite 200
Washington, DC 20024   Telephone 202-479-6984

National Alliance for Caregiving
7201 Wisconsin Avenue, Suite 620
Bethesda, MD 20814   Telephone 301-718-8444

National Association of Professional
Geriatric Care Managers
1604 North Country Club Road
Tucson, AZ 85716   Telephone 520-881-8008

National Autism Hotline
Autism Services Center
Prichard Building
605 9th Street, P. O. Box 507
Huntington, WV 25710   Telephone 304-525-8014

National Cancer Institute
Cancer Information Service
9000 Rockville Pike
Bethesda, MD 20892   Telephone 800-422-6237

National Caregiving Foundation
401 Wythe Street, Suite A-3
Alexandria, VA 22314   Telephone 800-930-1357

National Center for Home Equity Conversion (NCHEC)
7373 147th Street W, Suite 115
Apple Valley, MN 55124   Telephone 612-953-4474

National Children's Cancer Society
1015 Locust Street, Suite 1040
St. Louis, MO 63101   Telephone 800-532-6459

National Clearinghouse for Legal Services, Inc.
205 West Monroe Street, 2nd Floor
Chicago, IL 60606-5013   Telephone 312-263-3830

National Coalition for Cancer Survivorship (NCCS)
1010 Wayne Avenue, Suite 505
Silver Spring, MD 20910   Telephone 301-650-8868

National Committee for the Prevention
Of Elder Abuse
Medical Center of Central Massachusetts
119 Belmont Street
Worcester, MA 01605   Telephone 508-793-6166

National Council on Aging
409 3rd Street, SW, 2nd Floor
Washington, DC 20004   Telephone 202-479-1200

National Family Caregivers Association
9621 East Bexhill Drive
Kensington, MD 20895   Telephone 800-896-3650

National Fathers Network
Kindering Center
16120 NE 8th Street
Bellevue, WA 98008   Telephone 206-747-4004

National Federation of Interfaith
Volunteer Caregivers, Inc.
368 Broadway, Suite 103, P.O. Box 1939
Kingston, NY 12401   Telephone 800-350-7438

National Easter Seal Society
230 W. Monroe Street, #1800
Chicago, IL 60606   Telephone 800-221-6827

National Hospice Organization
1901 N. Moore Street, Suite 901
Arlington, VA 22209   Telephone 800-658-8898

National Insurance Consumer Helpline   Telephone 800-942-4242

National Organization of Social Security
Claimants Representatives
6 Prospect Street
Midland Park, NJ 07432   Telephone 201-444-1415

National Meals on Wheels Foundation
22675 44th Street SW, #305
Grand Rapids, MI 49509   Telephone 800-999-6262

National Multiple Sclerosis Society
733 Third Avenue
New York, NY 10017   Telephone 800-344-4867

National Organization for Rare Disorders
100 Route 37, P.O. Box 8923
New Fairfield, CT 06812   Telephone 800-999-6673

National Respite Locator Service
800 Eastowne Drive, Suite 105
Chapel Hill, NC 27514-2204   Telephone 800-773-5433

National Spinal Cord Injury Hotline
2200 N. Forest Park Avenue
Baltimore, MD 21207   Telephone 800-526-3456

National Self-Help Clearinghouse
(Provides referrals to support groups)
25 W. 43rd Street, Room 620
New York, NY 10036   Telephone 212-354-8525

National Stroke Association
8480 E. Orchard Road, Suite 1000
Englewood, CO 80111   Telephone 800-787-6537

O

P
Paralyzed Veterans of America
801 18th Street, NW
Washington, DC 20006-3715   Telephone 202-416-7622

Parents Helping Parents
The Family Resource Center
3041 Olcott Street
Santa Clara, CA 95054   Telephone 408-727-5775

Pharmaceutical Research and
Manufacturers of America (PhRMA)
1100 15th Street, NW
Washington, DC 20005   Telephone 800-762-4636

Q

R

Range Respite
302 Chestnut Street, Suite 302
Virginia, MN 55792   Telephone 218-749-5051

Resource Director for Older People
National Institute on Aging
Public Information Office
9000 Rockville Pike, Building 31
Bethesda, MD 20892   Telephone 800-222-2225

Respitality
United Cerebral Palsy
80 Whitney Street
Hartford, CT 06150   Telephone 860-236-6201

S

Shepherd's Centers of America
6700 Troost, Suite 616
Kansas City, MO 64131   Telephone 800-547-7073

Special Kids, Special Families
415201 Village Green Boulevard
Canton, MI 48187   Telephone 313-481-0008

Stroke Connection
7272 Greenville Avenue
Dallas, TX 75231-4596   Telephone 800-553-6321

T

Texas Respite Resource Network
P. O. Box 7330/519
West Houston Street
San Antonio, TX 78207-0330 Telephone 210-228-2794

Time Out Respite and Home Support Program
1601 Broad Street, Room 206
Philadelphia, PA 19122 Telephone 215-204-6540

U

United Cerebral Palsy Association, Inc. (UCPA)
1660 "L" Street, NW, Suite 700
Washington, DC 20036 Telephone 800-872-5827

United Parkinson Foundation
833 W. Washington Boulevard
Chicago, IL 60607 Telephone 312-733-1893

United Seniors Health Cooperative
1331 "H" Street, NW, Suite 500
Washington, DC 20005-4706 Telephone 202-393-6222

US Too! International, Inc.
(Support network for caregivers and
loved ones with prostate cancer)
930 North York Road, Suite 50
Hinsdale, IL 60521-2993 Telephone 800-808-7866

V

W
Well Spouse Foundation
610 Lexington Avenue, Suite 8145
New York, NY 10022-6005   Telephone 800-838-0879

X

Y
Y-ME
National Breast Cancer Organization
212 West Van Buren, 5th Floor
Chicago, IL 60607   Telephone 800-221-2141

Z
Zenith Health Care
(Assistance to caregivers of people
with Alzheimer's Disease)
245 S. El Molino Boulevard
Pasadena, CA 91101   Telephone 818-831-4024

References

Agel, Jerome and Glanze, Walter D (Ed.). *Pearls of Wisdom, A Harvest of Quotations from All Ages,* Harper Perennial, 1987.

Llardo, Joseph, Ph.D., L.C.S.W. and Rothman, Carole R., Ph.D., *I'll Take Care of You,* New Harbinger Publications, Inc., 1999.

Babcock, Elise Needell. *When Life Becomes Precious,* Bantam Books, 1997.

Brandt, Avrene L. *Caregiver's Reprieve,* Impact Publishers, 1998.

Burton, Scott. *A Life in the Balance,* Inconvenience Productions, 1997.

Callanan, Maggie and Kelley, Patricia. *Final Gifts,* Bantam Books, 1992.

Cook, John. *The Book of Positive Quotations,* Fairview Press, 1993.

Dollinger, Malin, M.D., Rosenbaum, Ernest H., M.D. and Cable, Greg. *Everyone's Guide to Cancer Therapy,* Somerville House Books Limited. 1994.

Freeman, Angela Beasley. *100 Years of Women's Wisdom, Timeless Insights from Great Women of the Twentieth Century,* Walnut Grove Press, 1999.

Longaker, Christine. *Facing Death and Finding Hope,* Doubleday, 1997.

LeVert, Susan. *When Someone You Love Has Cancer,* Dell Publishing, 1995.

ASSOCIATIONS

American Cancer Society

Cancer Care, Inc.

Inland Hospice Association

Leukemia Society of America

National Cancer Institute

WebofCare.com, Inc.

Index

Printed in the United States
123221LV00002B/1-273/A